HOW TO CHEAT ON YOUR DIET

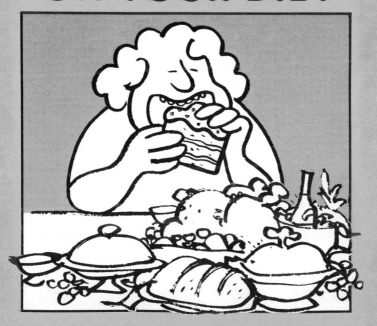

By H.R. BULLOCK • Illustrated by ROY McKIE

PRICE/STERN/SLOAN
Publishers, Inc., Los Angeles
1983

T3-BOR-541

The material in this book has been excerpted from
The Fat Book published by Price/Stern/Sloan Publishers, Inc.

Copyright© 1979, 1983 by H.R. Bullock
Illustrations Copyright© 1979 by Price/Stern/Sloan Publishers, Inc.
Published by Price/Stern/Sloan Publishers, Inc.
410 North La Cienega Boulevard, Los Angeles, California 90048

Printed in the United States of America. All rights reserved. No part of this
publication may be reproduced, stored in a retrieval system, or transmitted,
in any form or by any means, electronic, mechanical, photocopying, record-
ing, or otherwise, without the prior written permission of the publishers.

ISBN: 0-8431-1032-5
PSS! is a registered trademark of Price/Stern/Sloan Publishers, Inc.

HOW TO USE
THIS BOOK

Constructive, creative diet-cheating
requires only one thing: TOTAL BELIEF:

These guilt-free alibis have been devised by
ingenious Happy Heavies. They work!

BUT ONLY PROVIDING YOU
ABSOLUTELY BELIEVE YOU ARE NOT
CHEATING. NOT EVEN A TINY BIT!
(Which, of course, you're not.)

CAKE EATEN OVER A SINK DOESN'T COUNT

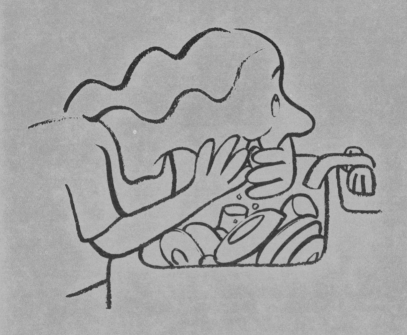

Your stomach is used to working in the dining room.
When you eat anywhere else, it's busy with other
things and won't notice.

AFTER YOU PUT SACCHARINE IN YOUR COFFEE, ANY DOUGHNUTS YOU DUNK ARE WITHOUT CALORIES, TOO!

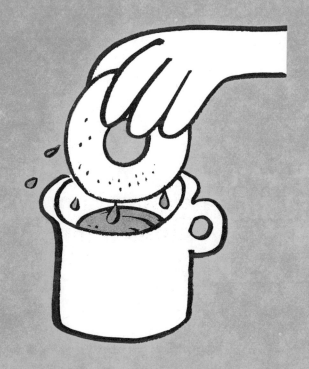

Saccharine is such a powerful artificial sweetener
it removes calories from anything it touches.

IF YOU'VE STAYED STRICTLY ON A DIET ALL DAY... A MIDNIGHT SNACK WON'T COUNT

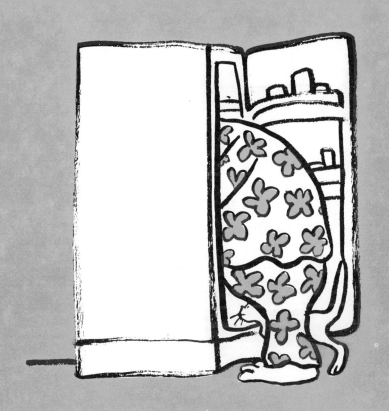

Your body has been so impressed by your will power
that its ability to absorb calories has shut down for
the night.

SAMPLE SNACKS HANDED OUT IN SUPERMARKETS DON'T COUNT

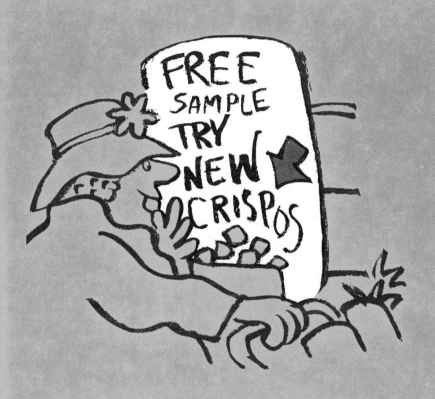

This can't have any calories because it isn't food, it's ADVERTISING. You wouldn't count it any more than if you ate the yellow pages.

FOOD EATEN IN THE DARK DOESN'T COUNT

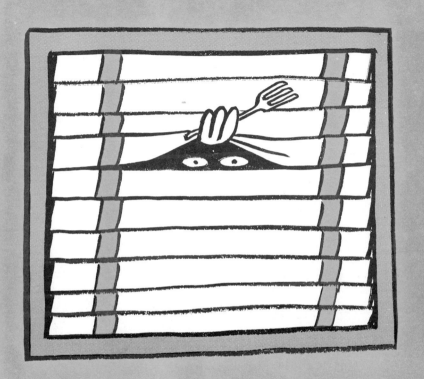

Any snacks polished off in a dark kitchen can neither be NOTED nor STORED up by the body. If there are no witnesses, nothing can be proved.

SNACK BAR FOOD
ORDERED JUST SO
YOU CAN REST YOUR
FEET DOESN'T COUNT

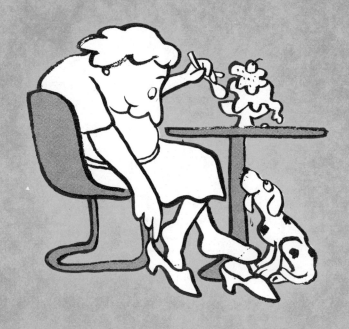

When you have to order food just to help another part of your body it's not like really eating. To sit there you HAVE to buy something. But it isn't food—more like a coin for a parking meter.

FOOD FROM SOMEONE ELSE'S PLATE DOESN'T COUNT

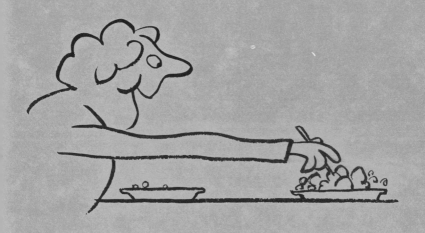

Since these portions were not intended for you they don't count against you. They count against the wasteful person who didn't clean the plate.

IF YOU LEAVE
SOMETHING ON YOUR
PLATE, THEN WHAT
YOU HAVE EATEN
WON'T COUNT VERY
MUCH

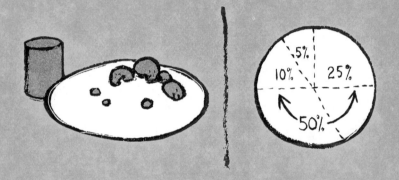

If you'd eaten EVERYTHING it would have been much worse. By eating LESS, you have demonstrated will power which means that what you ate shouldn't count AT ALL.

If this is confusing, let your accountant explain it.

NIBBLING ON LEFTOVERS YOU'RE TAKING OUT TO THE DOG DOESN'T COUNT

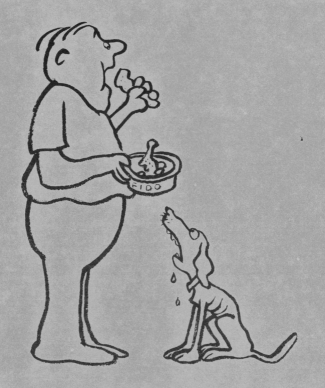

These items are clearly intended to give to your pet. Your body is NOT expecting them. If you take a few quick nibbles, it goes on Fido's record, NOT YOURS.

A SNACK WITH YOUR GLASSES OFF DOESN'T COUNT

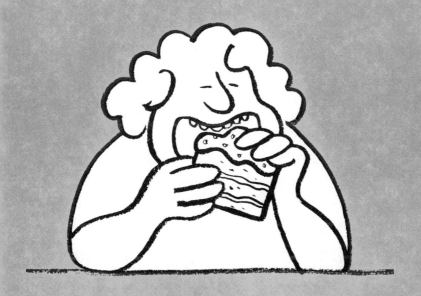

If you're not wearing corrective lenses, then when you take a nibble it is only registered VERY HAZILY on your senses. Not having a clear picture of exactly what's going on up there, your body will NOT regard the food as "definite intake," so you don't have to either.

A SNACK TAKEN ONLY TO HELP YOU GET TO SLEEP DOESN'T COUNT

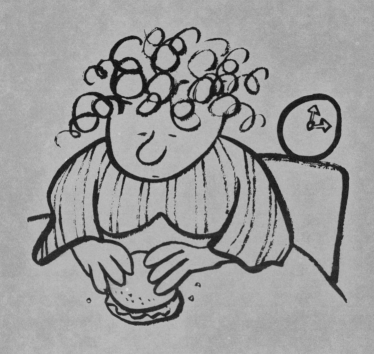

You are not using the snack as food but as a
PRESCRIPTION REMEDY to alleviate insomnia.
It's so much better for you than any knockout pills
that it should not be counted as food.

SAMPLES OF FOOD
BEING PREPARED
DON'T COUNT

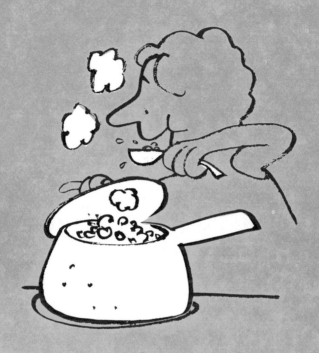

NEVER count nibbles taken ONLY TO FIND
OUT WHETHER FOOD IS PROPERLY
COOKED. No one should ever be penalized for
being conscientious over the correct nutrition of
their loved ones.

FOOD EATEN REALLY
REALLY FAST DOESN'T
COUNT

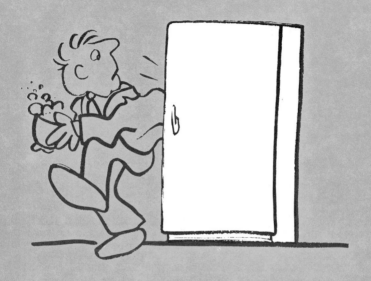

Whatever food you can get out of the refrigerator, eat, and then back in before the door automatically swings shut again DOES NOT COUNT AGAINST YOU EVEN A TINY BIT! Obviously this quick-gulped food is swallowed so fast you metabolism never gets a good grip on it.

GIFTS MEANT FOR ANOTHER DON'T COUNT

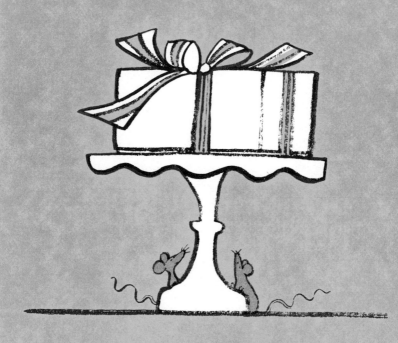

You can take free samples of any goodies given to somebody else, since the gift card clearly states all the calories are intended for THEM.

BUSINESS LUNCHES DON'T COUNT

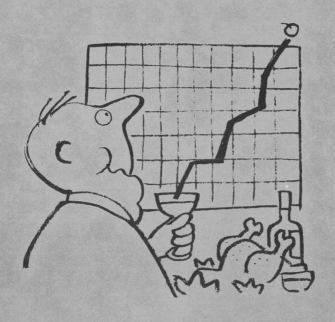

Meals consumed during the business day for business reasons are NOT a personal intake. They are a PROFESSIONAL OBLIGATION. In order to display an effective prosperous sincere image, you must order and consume extra courses and drinks. Dessert is necessary to give you more time to close that deal. All business lunches are as deductible from your diet as the bill is from your taxes.

ANYTHING EATEN ABSENT-MINDEDLY DOESN'T COUNT

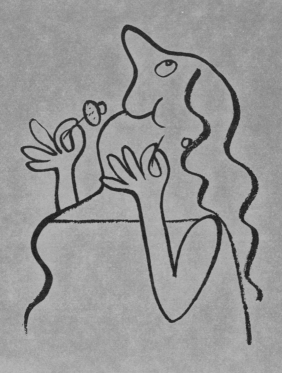

When your thoughts are far away, so is your digestive system. It cannot absorb anything received unconsciously.

FOOD EATEN AT CHURCH SUPPERS DOESN'T COUNT!

It would be blasphemous to label such blessed vittles as being for one's SELF. This is food for the SOUL, not the body.

SNACKS EATEN WHILE ON THE TELEPHONE DON'T COUNT!

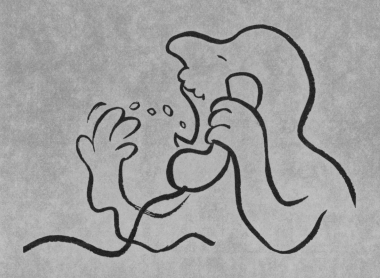

When concentrating on a telephone conversation, your senses of HEARING and THINKING take over your body. Your digestion is DORMANT, not expecting to receive anything while the throat is busy talking. So the snacks go right past it. This is true for both local and long distance conversations and even intercom calls, if tense enough.

FOOD BOUGHT FROM A CHARITY DOESN'T COUNT

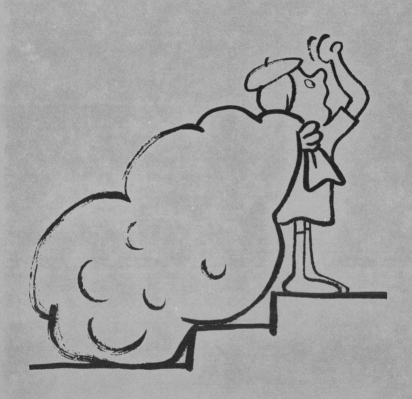

You can eat Girl Scout cookies without counting calories because they're not really food, they're a charitable contribution.

FOOD PREPARED FOR GUESTS WHO DIDN'T SHOW UP WON'T COUNT AGAINST YOU

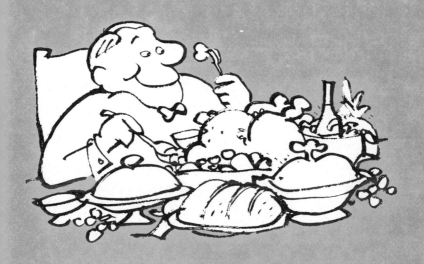

The food the guests didn't eat was clearly meant for THEM. So were the calories. Besides, by failing to show up, your guests have incurred a guilt/calorie debt which makes the food free if YOU eat it.

SOME FINAL QUICKIES:

- If you drink milk DIRECTLY FROM THE CARTON it doesn't count.

- *The jumbo size soft drinks don't count extra WHEN THEY'RE ON A SPECIAL SALE.*

- A midnight snack doesn't count if you're so tired there may be a chance you'll sleep through breakfast.

- Food consumed during an INTIMATE CANDLELIGHT SUPPER DOESN'T COUNT. This isn't starch, it's seduction.

- *Snacks eaten IDLY IN A DINER WHILE WAITING FOR SOMEONE ELSE don't count. You're only trying to avoid a loitering charge. It's a legal device, not a lunch.*

- Maple Syrup NEVER counts. It's a wood product. You wouldn't count toothpicks, would you?

NOW HAVE A BIG DAY!
YOU'RE ENTITLED

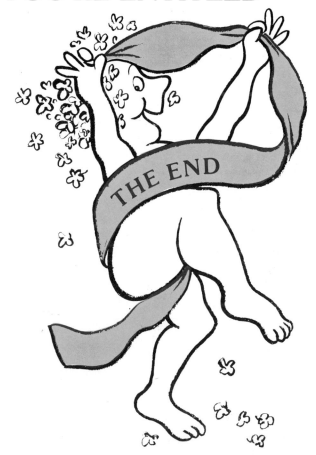

THE END

This book is published by

PRICE/STERN/SLOAN
Publishers, Inc., Los Angeles

whose other splendid titles include such literary classics as:

YOU KNOW YOU'RE OFF YOUR DIET WHEN . . .

THE ABSOLUTE TRUTH ABOUT MARRIAGE

BETS YOU CAN'T LOSE

MORE BETS YOU CAN'T LOSE

MINDTEASERS

HOW MANY 3-CENT STAMPS IN A DOZEN?

MORE THAN ENOUGH REASONS
TO HAVE SEX ANYTIME

and many, many more

They are available at $1.75 each wherever books are sold, or
may be ordered directly from the publisher by sending
check or money for the total amount plus $1.00 for
handling and mailing. For a complete list of titles
send a *stamped, self-addressed envelope* to:

PRICE/STERN/SLOAN   *Publishers, Inc.*
410 North La Cienega Boulevard, Los Angeles, California 90048

pss!®

WL091